HANGOVER GUIDEBOOK

EVERYTHING YOU NEED TO KNOW ABOUT HAVING FUN WITHOUT REGRETS THE NEXT DAY

TABLE OF CONTENTS

- INTRODUCTION 3
- CHAPTER ONE 9
- WHAT IS A HANGOVER? 9
- CHAPTER TWO 23
- HANGOVER; UNDERSTANDING OF ALCOHOL ITSELF 23
- CHAPTER THREE 41
- TIPS FOR AVOIDING A HANGOVER BEFORE THINGS GET WORSE! 41
- CHAPTER FOUR 44
- TREATING YOUR HANGOVER 44
- CHAPTER FIVE 52
- A GOOD HANGOVER CURE AND THE CURES TO AVOID 52
- CHAPTER SIX 60
- WHAT TO EAT WHEN YOU HAVE A HANGOVER? 60
- CONCLUSION 68

INTRODUCTION

No one enjoys a hangover. Known medically as "veisalgia" (a word that comes from two sources, interestingly-aglia, from the Greek for "pain," and the Norwegian word kveis, or "uneasiness following debauchery," it is a state universally disliked. And yet, despite this, we still don't know a lot about hangovers-what specifically causes them, for example, or what works to get rid of them. Certainly, the best way to prevent a hangover is to not drink at all, but if you are going to consume alcohol, how does one avoid feeling awful the next day?

Strangely enough, not a lot of research has been done on the hangover. While since 1965 many books have been published on the effects of alcohol, hundreds of those have focused specifically on the hangover.

Hangover usually is distinguished by patients complaining of nausea, headache, lack of sense of "well-being," intestinal distress such as diarrhea or inability to eat, tremulousness in the limbs, and decreased ability to perform jobs that deal with cognitive, visual, or spatial awareness or performance. The book makes clear that while hangovers are typically associated with the concept of alcoholism or those in need of alcohol treatment, most who suffer from hangovers are light or moderate drinkers-those less able to tolerate alcohol, in other words.

So how much alcohol must someone consume before he or she will have a hangover? The truth is we really don't know but we can estimate.

The study claims that for men, consuming "five to seven" cocktails (meaning standard cocktails, like a gin and tonic, not a massive "Hurricane" in New Orleans, for example) is nearly always followed by a hangover. And for women, that number is even smaller-women usually experience hangover symptoms after three to five standard cocktails, because they metabolize alcohol differently than men.

And yet, it seems that limiting one's drinking doesn't always prevent a hangover. Research has shown that hangovers are not solely caused by dose of alcohol, but sometimes by type. "Congeners" may partially be to blame.

Congeners are byproducts found in many darker types of liquor like whiskey, wine, tequila, and brandy, and may increase the severity of a hangover-as well as the frequency at which they occur. Clear alcohols such as light rum, gin, and vodka are less frequently the cause of hangovers, which may be a factor in severe alcoholics gravitating toward such potations rather than darker-colored drinks.

If you find yourself with a hangover, there's no silver bullet to cure it, sadly enough. But the common knowledge of hydration seems to be less effective than taking a small dose of vitamin B6 before, during, or after consuming alcohol. Definitely avoid Tylenol or any kind of acetaminophen when drinking however-the combination can cause liver damage.

This book is one of many resources designed to help those seeking an advanced approach to treatment for alcohol or drug abuse. Let's get started.

I am from Poland, we drink here a lot and we know how to cure hangover. If you wonder about Poland, what comes first to your mind is a lot of vodka or alcohol, it's true we drink a lot, and we have great ways to get rid of hangover, we know how to cure it.

REASON WHY WE NEED HELP

Poland has always faced the stereotype of having an above-average level of alcohol consumption. The current trend, however, serves as a red flag. While the majority of the European Union has seen a consistent decline in alcohol intake, rates increased by 30% in Poland between 2001 and 2012. This is in sharp contrast to the yearly decline in consumption the country had enjoyed since 1980.

The rising trend is more relevant than ever in Poland due to the concurrent increase in other factors like obesity and diabetes. Combining these risk factors may dramatically raise the number of hospitalizations over the next two decades. Alcohol-related hospital admissions due to short-term use include automobile accidents, coma, and even seizures in acute alcohol poisoning.

Chronic abuse leads to liver failure and shrinks the brain by destroying neurons.

Neurons are especially damaged in area that we use for planning and complex thinking. In the past, it was suggested that mild alcohol consumption could be beneficial to heart health. However, current research has found that even one glass of wine per night increases the risk of breast and other forms of cancer.

Alcohol abuse is a public health problem that may be on the rise in Poland. Having an educated population regarding the health effects of drinking may not stop abuse, but it can encourage discourse to reduce access to alcohol. Limiting access involves steps including heavier alcohol taxes or limitations on sales. In Russia, moves to reduce reduction were effective in reducing sales, but they also increased the production of more dangerous, illegally produced alcohols. In Canada, hard liquor can only be sold at certain government-run liquor stores. Not only are these stores limited in number, but they also close relatively early in the evening to discourage late night binge drinking.

Both of these countries still have alcoholics, and legislative change will not address the culture of drinking in Poland, but it is time to become more aggressive in policymaking. If you think you have a problem, talk to your doctor and see what options you have.

CHAPTER ONE
WHAT IS A HANGOVER?

Those dreaded hangovers are something people have been dealing with for thousands and thousands of years. However, many of those individuals never really figured out what was causing them...and neither do many people now. If a person was able to figure out just what causes a hangover, wouldn't it be fair to say that they can be eliminated almost completely? It's true. There are many ways to avoid them, but let's first look at how they are caused. First, a hangover is basically a series of unpleasant symptoms directly linked to the over-consumption of alcohol, as well as other substances and lack thereof (i.e. water). Most of us know the common symptoms including headaches, sensitivity to light and sound, irritability, grogginess and so on. But each of these symptoms are actually caused by contributions from many different things such as vitamin B12 deficiency, and lack of hydration. The symptoms can last from say an hour all the way into a few days for some people. Ouch!

Some of the main causes of a hangover are due to dehydration, drinking too many too fast, carbonated drinks, drinking on an empty stomach, congeners, acetaldehyde, vitamin B12 deficiency and more. We will go over the more apparent symptoms here.

Alcohol is a diuretic, which means it makes you urinate...regularly. This constant urination actually is one of the main causes of your headache in the morning. The headaches are often caused by dehydration. When you urinate often, you lose water. Many people forget to consume water when out drinking and this can lead to quite some pain the next day. Your body needs water in order to process to alcohol, so maybe try a glass between each beer. You and your body will both be happy later.

Drinking too much too fast or binge drinking obviously will cause a hangover due to the fact that your body can only process about a beer an hour. When you pile on three, four, or more beers in an hour, the toxins that your body turns the alcohol into run rampant until your body can properly metabolize it into non-toxic substances.

Many people already know that mixing drinks can lead to worsened hangovers. This is usually caused by mixing carbonated drinks with non-carbonated hard liquor drinks, also mixing lighter and darker colored drinks can lead to heavier hangovers due to the congener content. The sweeter drinks can fool a person, too. When you are drinking beers all night and someone hands you a lovely margarita, of course, you will drink it in a similar fashion as to that of your last beer.

Carbonated drinks such as champagne can speed up your hangover due to the fact that carbonated beverages speed up your body's metabolism. It takes a while for your body to adjust to a non-carbonated alcoholic drink and by the time you realize it, you are already feeling pretty nauseas. Think of it like the difference between digesting a salad and a steak. Which takes longer?

Next, we come to by-products of both fermentation and your own body's metabolism of alcohol. When alcohol is produced, many by-products of fermentation are produced. These are called congeners. They cause hangovers. The cheaper the drink, the less congener are taken out.

That is why you get worsened hangovers for drinking cheap liquor. Now as for your body, when you break down alcohol, an enzyme breaks it down into a toxic substance called acetaldehyde. Then it breaks it down with another enzyme into a non-toxic substance. When you have a lot of acetaldehyde in your body and your liver can't break it all down in time, it can assist in liver damage as well as get you pretty sick the next day. One thing to note is that in addition to acetaldehyde, acetaminophen can also damage your liver due to the fact that now you would be having two toxins up in your liver. That puts quite a bit of pressure on your liver and it can only handle so much. Acetaminophen is found in products such as Tylenol.

One thing to remember here is that it is a good thing to know what causes a hangover as it will show you the way to preventing the things from happening in the first place.

You might know what the definition of hangover is but how do the boffins define it? Sometimes, it's interesting to see what a dictionary would say about being having a hangover, or even a medical encyclopedia.

But rather than do that, I will translate the definition and symptoms into layman's language for you so you don't have to scratch your head in pain. After all, you might well have a headache now and wonder if you have all the classic hangover symptoms. You don't want to read any complicated words.

The most succinct definition of a hangover is this very interpretation.

The basic definition of a hangover

A hangover is a combination of unpleasant and disagreeable physical symptoms following heavy alcohol consumption.

Translation: A hangover is when you wake up feeling bad after drinking too much.

Symptoms of a hangover

These are the symptoms you suffer from when you have a hangover.

Headache - head hurts

Nausea - You feel like vomiting

Sensitivity to light and noise - The computer screen is burning holes through your eyes

Lethargy - Laziness and desire to stay all day in bed

Dysphoria - Feeling down

Diarrhea - Regular visits to the toilet

Thirst - A dry, parched mouth

Other symptoms of a hangover:

Weakness - Feeling tired and floppy

Sweating - The sheets are yellow

Halitosis - Nasty bad breath

Lack of concentration - You can't remember what you were talking about

Anxiety - Becoming stressed about small things

Symptoms of a hangover

How do you know when you have the very definition of a hangover? You have the classic hangover symptoms of course. Just in case you're confused, you can find out what hangover symptoms are. Knowing more about these may also help you better understand more about the causes of that morning after feeling?

1. Dryness of the mouth

Severe dehydration may wake you up with the driest mouth ever. So dry in fact that it sometimes feels like a sandpaper coated rat has slept in there, and your mouth attracts the dust and particles in the air while you sleep.

2. Horrible teeth

Your teeth have a coating of sugar from a drink from last night. Of course, you naturally forgot to brush them before sleeping too. Now run to the bathroom and clean them hard!

That might help your bad breath too, another hangover symptom that many people wake up with.

3. Hangover headache

We all know the pounding, thrashing, monster of a deathly headache, caused by the combination of a lack of vitamins & minerals, dehydration and possible congener's in your drink. This has to be the most painful of the hangover symptoms.

4. Bad stomach

Your stomach is feeling unstable and rebellious from last night's strong drinks on an empty stomach. It may make you vomit or you have diarrhea or both.

5. Red eyes

Your eyes can actually become dehydrated too, leaving them all red and veiny and looking smooth for that lunch date the next day with your new girl/boyfriend or his/her parents.

6. Tiredness

Given that excessive alcohol consumption means you don't actually sleep properly, at least for the first few hours after collapsing on your bed; it's hardly surprising you feel like you only slept 15 minutes. In addition to this, alcohol consumption can deplete your blood/sugar level, which can make you feel even more tired.

Pathology and possible remedies for hangover cure

As a dietary staple in cultures around the world, alcohol has been consumed widely for thousands of years. The ancient Egyptians worshiped a beer god who they believed invented the sacred beverage. Unfortunately, no god existed to protect them from the adverse effects of alcohol, collectively named a hangover.

Despite the amount of research into alcoholism and alcohol dependency, very little research has been conducted on hangovers and the causes of its associated symptoms. Perhaps the lack of attention is attributable to the moral hazard incurred by any discoveries or formulations found to prevent or treat hangovers. Many clinicians believe the hangover to be a deterrent to consuming large amounts of alcohol--some would rather a cure remains elusive. Although this belief has merit, the market for such a discovery, supported by double-blind clinical research, would be enormous. However, executing necessary research poses problems in of itself as procedures for such studies would be difficult to adhere to. It is no surprise that few clinical studies have been conducted to explore the effectiveness of existing remedies and formulations.

There are a few distinct theories behind the causes of hangover symptoms, although a combination of them all is the likely case. Two identifiable contributors to hangover symptoms are dehydration and acetaldehyde.

Alcohol is a diuretic, causing water loss within the body. When alcohol is consumed, it inhibits the release of the antidiuretic hormone (ADH) from the pituitary gland. This hormone regulates the body's re-absorption rate of water within the kidneys.

As alcohol interrupts the hormone levels, water reabsorption slows and more water is excreted from the body. This explains the numerous "bathroom breaks" one takes while consuming large amounts of alcohol. Although water is obtained from the alcoholic beverages themselves, a majority is ultimately expelled due to hormone disruption of ADH levels. In beverages with higher alcohol content, the impact is even more pronounced. For example, after consuming a glass of wine (12.5% alcohol by volume), well over 100% the amount in water will be released from the body.

Mild to moderate cases dehydration can result from an intake of alcohol. Symptoms of dehydration are similar to those experienced during a hangover: dry or sticky mouth, lightheadedness, headache, lethargy, and confusion. The cure for dehydration is an obvious one--water. To help prevent dehydration while drinking alcohol, glasses of water should be consumed intermittently. Extra care should be taken when drinking beverages with higher concentrations of alcohol as these intensify dehydration.

Electrolyte balance can also be disrupted due to water loss (alongside water-soluble B and C vitamins). Electrolytes can be replenished through sports beverages such as Gatorade and Vitamin Water.

Taking B-complex and vitamin C can help restore these levels within the body.

Acetaldehyde is identified as the major culprit contributing to hangovers. Acetaldehyde is a chemical compound produced during the metabolism of alcohol within the body. It is a toxic substance (much more than that of alcohol itself) that can produce a plethora of the symptoms experienced during a hangover. Its effects include flushing of the skin, throbbing headache, nausea, and vomiting.

When alcohol is consumed; it is initially broken down by the enzyme alcohol dehydrogenase, converting the alcohol into acetaldehyde. Acetaldehyde is then converted to acetic acid (vinegar) by the enzyme acetaldehyde dehydrogenase. This second stage requires sulfur-containing antioxidants in order to complete the conversion.

If antioxidant supplies are depleted during alcohol consumption, a buildup of acetaldehyde can result and escape into the bloodstream.

A build-up of acetaldehyde can wreak havoc on biological functions, inhibiting mitochondria reactions and ultimately causing hangover symptoms. This is seen in alcoholic patients undergoing treatment with the drug Disulfiram. Disulfiram prevents the conversion of acetaldehyde into acetic acid by blocking necessary enzyme function. Alcohol consumption while taking Disulfiram will result in amplified hangover symptoms--throbbing headache, nausea and vomiting, mental confusion and possibly circulatory failure--strong deterrents to alcohol consumption.

A potential cure for this buildup of acetaldehyde is supplementation with sulfur-containing antioxidants such as N-Acetyl-L-Cysteine (NAC). NAC is readily absorbed into the body and binds with acetaldehyde in its conversion process to acetic acid. This helps prevent antioxidant depletion and the toxic effects of acetaldehyde. NAC's antioxidant properties may also help protect against liver damage such as fatty liver disease. NAC can be readily purchased at most health-food stores and vitamin outlets.

Commercial formulations containing NAC and specifically designed for hangovers also exist.

Other theories explaining hangovers include congeners and alcohol withdrawal. Congeners are compounds found in certain types of alcohol and created during the fermentation process. Some evidence exists that these compounds can contribute to a hangover. More congeners are found in dark alcohols and red wines, explaining why people commonly target these beverages as hangover-conducing.

Costing billions of dollars in losses to businesses each year, hangovers inflict their damage both physically and financially. The hangover remains an elusive beast, lacking both adequate clinical study and significant research. Alcohol abstinence is always a choice, but one doubted to find many followers.

CHAPTER TWO
HANGOVER; UNDERSTANDING OF ALCOHOL ITSELF

During the course of the year, we find ourselves going to all kinds of events such as birthdays, office luncheons, annual holidays, parties, and special occasions where alcohol is being served. Oftentimes along with feasting we also consume too much alcohol. This is a ▢uick guide to alleviating or completely avoiding hangover symptoms through an understanding of alcohol itself, physiological changes related to alcohol consumption, and a variety of suggested remedies for specific hangover symptoms.

Warning: First and foremost let me at least mention that you should always try to drink responsibly and arrange having a designated driver if you will be using your personal vehicle for transportation.

Classes of alcoholic beverages

Alcoholic beverages are divided into three general classes: beers, wines, and spirits. Beer and wine are produced by fermentation of sugar- or starch-containing plant material.

Beverages produced by fermentation followed by distillation have higher alcohol content and are known as liquor or spirits. The alcoholic strength of beer is usually 4% to 6% alcohol by volume (ABV), but it may be less than 2% or greater than 25%. Beers having an ABV of 60% (120 proof) have been produced by freezing brewed beer and removing water in the form of ice, a process referred to as "ice distilling". Beer is part of the drinking culture of various nations and has ac uired social traditions such as beer festivals, pub games, and pub crawling (sometimes known as bar hopping).

Wine is produced from grapes, and from fruits such as plums, cherries, or apples. Wine involves a longer fermentation process than beer and also a long aging process (months or years), resulting in an alcohol content of 9%-16% ABV. Sparkling wine can be made by means of a secondary fermentation. Fortified wine is wine (such as port or sherry), to which a distilled beverage (usually brandy) has been added.

Unsweetened, distilled, alcoholic beverages that have an alcohol content of at least 20% ABV are called spirits. Spirits are produced by the distillation of a fermented base product. Distilling concentrates the alcohol. For the most common distilled beverages, such as whiskey and vodka, the alcohol content is around 40%. Spirits can be added to wines to create fortified wines, such as port and sherry.

A 2009 study provided evidence that darker-colored liquors, such as bourbon, cause worse hangovers than lighter-colored liquors, such as vodka. The higher amount of "congeners" found in darker liquors compared to lighter ones was indicated as the cause. Studies that attempt to compare hangover producing potential and hangover severity of different alcoholic drinks suggest the following ordering (starting with the least hangover-inducing):

Distilled ethanol diluted in fruit juice, beer, vodka, gin, white wine, whiskey, rum, red wine, and brandy.

Alcohol and its effects, the basics.

Now let's cover some basics about alcohol. What is alcohol? Alcohol is a distilled or fermented beverage that transforms a grain, fruit, vegetable, or wood into ethanol. Ethanol, glucose, and sucrose are all in the same group of alcohols. Ethanol is the most common form of alcohol one finds in alcoholic beverages.

Alcohol is a psychoactive drug that has a depressant effect. Alcohol also stimulates insulin production, which speeds up glucose metabolism and can result in low blood sugar, causing irritability and (for diabetics) possible death. Alcohol intoxication affects the brain and causing symptoms such as slurred speech, delayed reflexes, vomiting or unconsciousness. Alcohol also limits the production of vasopressin (ADH) from the hypothalamus and the secretion of this hormone from the posterior pituitary gland. This is what causes the intense thirst that goes along with a hangover.

Now when alcohol builds up in the bloodstream faster than it can be metabolized by the liver, we enter a physiological state known as drunkenness or inebriation.

Alcohol is metabolized by a normal liver at the rate of about one ounce (one two-ounce shot of spirits, a normal beer, a regular sized glass of wine) every 90 minutes. An "abnormal" liver with conditions such as hepatitis, cirrhosis, gallbladder disease, and cancer will have a slower rate of metabolism.

Ethanol's acute effects are largely due to its nature as a central nervous system depressant and are dependent on blood alcohol concentrations. Here's a breakdown of what effects one can expect to experience from alcohol consumption according to the ▢uantity you consume:

20-99 mg/dL - Impaired coordination and euphoria

100-199 mg/dL - Ataxia, poor judgment, labile mood

200-299 mg/dL - Marked ataxia, slurred speech, poor judgment, labile mood, nausea, and vomiting

300-399 mg/dL - Stage 1 anesthesia, memory lapse, labile mood

400+ mg/dL - Respiratory failure, coma

In addition to respiratory failure and accidents caused by effects on the central nervous system, alcohol causes significant metabolic derangements. Hypoglycemia occurs due to ethanol's inhibition of gluconeogenesis, especially in children, and may cause lactic acidosis, ketoacidosis, and acute renal failure.

Some effects of alcohol intoxication are central to alcohol's desirability as a beverage. For example, some desirable effects from small quantities of alcohol consumption are euphoria and lowered social inhibitions. Other symptoms include slurred speech, impaired balance, loss of muscle coordination (ataxia), flushed face, dehydration, vomiting, reddened eyes, and erratic behavior. Other effects are unpleasant or dangerous because alcohol affects many different areas of the body at once.

This last point, the fact that alcohol affects many different areas of the body at once, is crucial to understanding the nature of a hangover. Why? Because everyone experiences different symptoms from their hangover, each hangover has to be dealt with individually. Here are 2 reasons underlying hangovers with completely different characteristics.

Many people from East Asian descent have a mutation in their genes that cause them to suffer from alcohol flush reaction, in which acetaldehyde accumulates after drinking, leading to immediate and severe hangover symptoms. Because for them a little alcohol goes a long way, they are also less likely to become alcoholics.

Older people report that their hangovers grow worse as they age. This is caused by declining supplies of alcohol dehydrogenase, the enzyme involved in metabolizing alcohol.

So what we've come to is the fact that there is currently no empirical proof for hangover prevention except reducing the amount of ethanol consumed or waiting for the body to metabolize the alcohol ingested.

This only happens when the liver oxidizes the alcohol. So what this means is that the most effective way to avoid any of the symptoms of an alcohol-induced hangover is to control or avoid drinking. Thus, no two hangovers are the same.

The physiology of a hangover

Excessive consumption of alcohol causes a delayed effect called a hangover. The hangover starts after the euphoric effects of ethanol have subsided. Hypoglycemia, dehydration, acetaldehyde intoxication, and glutamine rebound are all theorized causes of hangover symptoms. Hangover symptoms may persist for several days after alcohol was last consumed. Some aspects of a hangover are even viewed as symptoms of acute ethanol withdrawal, similar to the longer-duration effects of withdrawal from alcoholism.

Because alcohol impairs the ability of the liver to compensate for a drop in blood glucose levels, especially for the brain, it can result in the depletion of the liver's supply of glutathione, a detoxification agent, reducing its ability to effectively remove alcohol and its byproducts from the bloodstream. Since glucose is the primary energy source of the brain, this lack of glucose (hypoglycemia) contributes to symptoms such as fatigue, weakness, mood disturbances, and decreased attention and concentration related to a hangover.

The human body is a system of systems so physiological changes in one system change others. That's why the best approach is to try to handle several symptoms by resolving alcohol-related issues in multiple body systems simultaneously. For example, when you ingest alcohol, the salivary glands secrete enzymes to combine with the alcoholic beverage to make it more suitable for processing in the stomach and intestines. As the alcohol circulates throughout the digestive system and bloodstream it moves from one system to another. Just one drink affects the central nervous system, the digestive system, the endocrine system, the muscular system, the immune system, and the respiratory system, so with each additional drink, the effects compound and the potential dangers increase.

Because the alcohol moves around in the body rather than remaining in an organ, region, or system, it produces a wide range of negative physiological effects.

The most commonly reported characteristics of a hangover include headache, nausea, sensitivity to light and noise, lethargy, dehydration, fatigue, body aches, vomiting, diarrhea, flatulence, weakness, elevated body temperature and heart rate, hypersalivation, difficulty concentrating, sweating, anxiety, irritability, erratic motor functions (including tremor), trouble sleeping, severe hunger, halitosis, and lack of depth perception. Many people will also be repulsed by the thought, taste or smell of alcohol during a hangover. The symptoms vary significantly from person to person, and it is not clear whether hangovers directly affect cognitive abilities. The effects of a hangover subside over time.

Just as with lesser cases of low alcohol consumption, cases, where excessive amounts of alcohol have been consumed such as with alcohol poisoning treatment, strives to stabilize the patient and maintain a clear airway and respiration, while waiting for the alcohol to metabolize. In general, healthcare professionals will provide treatment for hypoglycemia (low blood sugar) with 50ml of 50% dextrose solution and saline flush, administer the vitamin thiamine to prevent seizure, check electrolytes to guide fluid replacement, apply hemodialysis (blood transfusion)if the blood concentration is dangerously high, or provide oxygen therapy.

Ineffective or unproven remedies

Recommendations for foods, drinks, and activities to relieve hangover symptoms abound, here are some that have been found to be ineffective or unproven.

The "Prairie Oyster" restorative, introduced at the 1878 Paris World Exposition, calls for raw egg yolk mixed with Worcestershire sauce, Tabasco sauce, salt, and pepper.

And in 1938, the Ritz-Carlton Hotel provided a hangover remedy in the form of a mixture of cola and milk.

By some accounts, cola beverages are believed to have been invented as a hangover remedy.

Alcoholic writer Ernest Hemingway relied on tomato juice and beer.

The "Black Velvet" consists of equal parts champagne and flat Guinness Stout.

A 1957 survey by a Wayne State University folklorist found widespread belief in the efficacy of heavy fried foods, tomato juice, and sexual activity.

Activities said to be restorative include a shower-alternating very hot and very cold water, exercise, and steam bath or sauna (although medical opinion holds this to be very dangerous, as the combination of alcohol and hyperthermia increases the likelihood of dangerous cardiac arrhythmias).

A 1976 research came to the conclusion that "The results indicate that both fructose and glucose effectively inhibit the metabolic disturbances induced by ethanol but they do not affect the symptoms or signs of alcohol intoxication and hangover." Nevertheless, consumption of honey (a significant fructose and glucose source) is often suggested as a way to reduce some of the effects of hangover.

Food and alcohol metabolism

Studies have found that when food is eaten before drinking alcohol, alcohol absorption is reduced and the rate at which alcohol is eliminated from the blood is increased. The mechanism for the faster alcohol elimination appears to be unrelated to the type of food. The likely mechanism is food-induced increases in alcohol-metabolizing enzymes and liver blood flow.

While this may not decrease your chances for getting a hangover, it's a good idea to eat before you drink, but know that doing so will eliminate the alcohol from your system faster than normal.

Scientifically based remedies

Earlier I said that because alcohol affects many different areas of the body at once, each hangover has to be dealt with individually. Why? Because everyone experiences different symptoms from their hangover, different from everyone else, and even from one state of drunkenness compared to another time of drunkenness. So the conclusion here is that there is currently no empirical proof for hangover prevention except reducing the amount of ethanol consumed or waiting for the body to metabolize the alcohol ingested. What this means is that the most effective way to avoid any of the symptoms of an alcohol-induced hangover is to control or avoid drinking.

But what are we supposed to do if we get a hangover? Sometimes it's not possible to wait for the effects of the hangover to wear off while coping with the symptoms. We need a way to effectively deal with this situation. You're right, we do. Here's the realization I've come to about how to handle the symptoms of a hangover.

The primary realization is that a hangover is not a thing, instead, it's a series of symptoms related to excessive alcohol consumption. That's key.

The second important point is that in order to deal with anyone hangover experience effectively you have to deal with the exact symptoms you're going through during a specific hangover.

Although there are many common symptoms experienced by most people routinely, sometimes new symptoms appear that were never part of previous hangovers. This is why it's best to handle the symptoms vs. trying to recover from a "hangover."

So below is a list of practices, substances, and products that deal with specific symptoms that should help you fight the effects of hangover whenever they occur.

You may also want to go back and re-read this chapter as there were remedies - such as eating before drinking, timing one's intake per ounce of ingestion, and preventing vomiting by abstinence in order to protect the stomach lining from erosion by alcohol - mentioned earlier that will not appear in this list.

1. Rehydration: Effective interventions include rehydration, prostaglandin inhibitors, and vitamin B6.

2. Milk thistle: A small dosage before and after alcohol consumption has been found to alleviate the some of the effects of a hangover such as

headaches, sluggishness, and nausea. Milk thistle works to regenerate liver cells and when combined with an excessive vitamin D intake from the sun, subjects have experienced rapidly decreasing hangover effects.

3. Tolfenamic acid is useful for nausea, vomiting, irritation, tremor, thirst, and dryness of mouth.

4. Vitamin B6 (pyritinol) can help to reduce some, but not all, of the symptoms of hangovers. For this Brewers' yeast or a B6 supplement are recommended.

5. Chlormethiazole was found to lower blood pressure and adrenaline output and, furthermore, to relieve unpleasant physical symptoms, but did not affect fatigue and drowsiness. Subjects with severe subjective hangover seemed to benefit more from the chlormethiazole treatment than subjects with a mild hangover.

6. Pedialyte may be an effective remedy for hangovers due to its replacement of lost electrolytes.

7. Candy or sugar: To raise lowered blood sugar levels caused by alcohol intake. Other options for

sweeteners to use are honey, brown sugar, maple syrup, agave nectar, and fructose.

8. Alcohol: There is a belief that consumption of additional alcohol in decreasing quantity over a period of hour's after the onset of a hangover will relieve symptoms. This is based upon the theory that the hangover represents a form of withdrawal and that by satiating the bodies need for alcohol the symptoms will be relieved. Certainly, the additional alcohol has a sedating and anesthetic effect, which also helps with symptoms.

The professional medical opinion holds that the practice merely postpones the symptoms, and courts alcohol dependence and addiction.

9. Medical marijuana: It is commonly believed that THC, the active chemical in marijuana, is an effective hangover remedy. THC may help ease the main symptoms of hangovers: nausea and headache. The advantage is two-fold; as once a sufferer's nausea has abated, and his appetite is stimulated, hypoglycemia becomes easier to resolve.

10. A traditional hangover remedy from India is to drink coconut water for the natural electrolytes which will assist in rehydration.

11. Acetyl-leucine sold under the brand name of Tanganil is believed to help pull you out of the "whirling pit" or spinning sensation felt by people under the influence of alcohol. This is caused by a dysfunction between the nerves which control the notion of balance in the ears and the brain. Tanganil is the standard remedy prescribed to people suffering from chronic vertigo.

12. Oxygen: There have been anecdotal reports from those with easy access to a breathing oxygen supply - medical staff, SCUBA divers and military pilots - that oxygen can also reduce the symptoms of hangovers caused by alcohol consumption. The theory is that the increased oxygen flow resulting from oxygen therapy improves the metabolic rate, and thus increases the speed at which toxins are broken down.

CHAPTER THREE
TIPS FOR AVOIDING A HANGOVER BEFORE THINGS GET WORSE!

We are often advised that drinking in moderation is the only choice for avoiding a hangover. How often have you stopped yourself from drinking more just because you hate the hangover symptoms next morning? Of course, alcohol consumption is not good for health and we know that. But sometimes such circumstances occur where we end up drinking more than we thought and meet our unwelcome friend, hangover.

The good news is that hangover can both be avoided as well as cured. You will have to figure out which is the best hangover remedy for you, and you surely have many options to try. Water is the first remedy to start with. Whether it is headache, sick feeling in the stomach or lethargy, water is the simplest option to try. Dehydration is often a symptom of hangover so consuming water as well as other fluids works really well. Water helps in flushing out the toxins developed in the body due to alcohol breakdown.

Nutrient depletion is also one of the side effects of alcohol consumption. Lack of essential vitamins and minerals is often responsible for the symptoms of hangover. Intake of good quality health supplements is also a hangover cure. You may want to include a multivitamin to your daily routine. You can also take good quality vitamin B and C tablets before drinking to avoid a hangover. If you are experiencing hangover symptoms, remember to eat something light and healthy. This way, your body gets enough resources to deal with the hangover and does not have to overexert with the digestion process.

Consuming food and other snacks while drinking are also ways of avoiding a hangover. When alcohol is consumed on empty stomach it is most harmful. If you are prone to alcohol, do some homework and find out which types of alcoholic drinks suit you. Avoid cocktails, carbonated drinks and sweetened forms of alcohol. Don't go for cheap beer or other alcoholic beverage. Big brands have better quality checks on the alcohol and it is less harmful. Also avoid bourbon, red wine and other dark drinks in excess.

Aspirin has been popularly used as a hangover remedy, but research finds it to be harmful. There is already enough irritation in your body and Aspirin does not bring it down. In fact, it can irritate the stomach even further. Aspirin is known to slow down metabolism which does not let you get rid of the alcohol and also makes you lethargic. Other pain relief tablets are also known to damage the liver so be careful while taking any of those.

Here is one piece of information that will allow you to prevent a hangover. Our body can absorb about 20ml of alcohol in one full hour. Drink slowly and include activities like food and talking with friends to slow you down. Taking a few precautions is better than a lot of hangover cure later. It is wiser to be careful and enjoy your drinks while still being healthy and ready for life later.

Drinking does not necessarily have to result in a hangover. There are many options available to avoid a hangover.

CHAPTER FOUR
TREATING YOUR HANGOVER

Rather than treating your hangover with a cure the next day, you may have realized that the best way to avoid getting hangover is simply to prevent it rather than waiting until you the next day when the pain is already there.

The unfortunate truth is that many of us forget to take a vitamin drink or to have the right amounts of water, fruit juice, and food after drinking and before sleeping in order to prevent their hangovers.

Why do we forget? Maybe something to do with a slight overindulgence the night before? Despite leaving the multivitamin effervescent pill with liver protection tint on the pillow so we do forget to take it, the fact is that in our inebriated state, we do sometimes forget, contrary to all the great advice that people give us about how hangovers can be prevented by taking an effervescent multivitamin before sleeping and/or eating a starchy meal after drinking.

We know it's much better and more effective to prevent hangovers rather than waiting until we are already hangover the next day.

However, every single drinker can forget and wake up feeling like donkey dung, no matter how clever they are.

Treating a hangover isn't a simple matter and finding the right cure for your evil, poisonous condition can be a challenge as we all know. If you're aware of the different levels of hangover you can suffer from, you'll probably be looking to match your condition up with the correct remedy or cure. So for treating each type of hangover the morning after kindly greets you with, we have listed a number of remedies for you:

1. Next day buzz

The next day buzz is hardly a real hangover. You'll maybe get away with drinking an espresso coffee and water. Yes, coffee is not generally recommended for hangovers, but this time you can give it a go-to wake you up as it won't dehydrate you too much, hopefully.

Pop a vitamin drink too and enjoy your lunch.

2. Gas head

Tired and unable to think too straight or concentrate for too long, you need a bit more of a pickup for treating your languid state.

Drink lots of fruit juice throughout the day and have a multivitamin. Make sure the foods you eat are starch-based like pasta and toast and maybe have a banana. Don't eat too much otherwise you may fall asleep.

A sports drink can also hydrate you nicely and pick you up when you're feeling like this.

3. The classic

To remind you of how you feel:

You still feel a bit drunk the next morning and have a classic next day headache, dry mouth and your guts are moving around a bit. You cannot concentrate and are continually drinking water, although you don't need the toilet.

Hmmm. The recommendation for treating this type of hangover is:

Eggs and bacon

2 bananas

Lots of water and fruit juice throughout the day

An energy drink without caffeine (sports drink)

4. The beast

Now we're talking. You really overloaded last night if you're suffering from The Beast today. A bee stung your brain, your breath is worse than the dog who just ate a 2-week old steak he found in a bin in the street and you feel like you'll vomit if you even think about alcohol. You're never going to drink again, ever. Well, until Friday maybe.

A tough, delicate condition to overcome.

To get back on track, you need:

Fruit juices, banana juice, and tomato juice tend to be very effective

Sugar drinks, (like soda) to rehydrate & increase your blood sugar level

When you can handle it, eat a banana with honey on it

Big multivitamin pill (preferably effervescent)

Have a hot shower or a bath to sweat out some alcohol, then blast cold water on your face and on your head

A brisk walk and some fresh air

Try to resist having a painkiller unless your head is really still unbearably painful, even after drinking and eating all. If it's really hard, pop an ibuprofen, but not a Tylenol as it can be tough on the liver after alcohol.

5. The daddy of all hangovers

If your hangover is any worse than the beast, you must have the Daddy of all hangovers. We feel very sorry for you and we understand what you're going through. As far as a cure goes, you'll just have to stay put, drinking water or sugar drinks before you can stomach anything solid. Try to sleep through the pain.

This is daddy of all hangovers personified, the very essence of the wicked witch of the pounding, shaking, cringing most terrible of aftershocks. You are a complete, gibbering, sweating, shivering mess and will be until next week unless you do something about it.

Everyone's been there, even the most conservative of teetotallers who think having 2 beers in one night is being a bit crazy. Yes, that boy with the square glasses and the green cardigan from the library who acts like he's 45 when he's only 21 has been there too. Probably.

The window to your room is fast shut, the air is stuffy and you've sucked all the oxygen out. Through your slitty, half closed, puffy eyes, you vaguely remember starting off the night on red wine, even though you hardly ever drink it, and you have a fuzzy recollection of some club which you don't have a clue about, at some point in the night, somewhere. That's all. Except you have no idea how you got back into your bed whatsoever.

Trouble avoided at least you think! Great, I'm safe, back and didn't have a fight, end up in a cell or wake up next to a cave troll! Bingo.

Yet about this time, your body's simultaneously telling you something's up - some dark, evil, bubbling potion that passed by your lips is now starting to take its poisonous toll on your head and stomach. Right now as you open those puffy eyes.

You start to wonder if a bear came along while you were sleeping before you even open your eyes to painful shards of light at around 10 am, after only 6 hours sleep.

Not only that, the same bear has then proceeded to jump on your head in the night and boot you in the stomach a few times before stuffing its furry paw down your throat and leaving it there all night.

The headache hits you like your head just got clapped between two ancient Roman gongs when you get up to go to the toilet! You think you're going to blow chunks; you just make it, but stagger back to bed and try to get back to sleep to get through it. No way!

Any attempt at drinking water or eating and you just vomit. This is one bad momma. Instead of getting better, an hour later you feel even worse!

This time, it seems like only a flat drink of a sugar soda drink and a painkiller (preferably ibuprofen) can do to kill the evil head pains and make eating and drinking bearable. Then, just stay in bed and drink water and a vitamin detox and eat when you're ready to stomach it. It may take a few hours, that's all. Once you feel able to get up, have a hot bath or go for a walk and eat something, to help your body process the alcohol out faster.

CHAPTER FIVE
A GOOD HANGOVER CURE AND THE CURES TO AVOID

A good hangover cure is the key difference between having a productive, relatively painless and even enjoyable day and having a grim, wasteful and useless day in bed with severe pain and nausea. So how do you get relief fast and even better, avoid medication that could be bad for your liver?

And how do you boost your body's natural ability to get rid of a hangover faster for the next time? These tips and techniques can help you.

1. Prevent hangovers using a vitamin kit

Preventing hangovers is much, much more effective than desperately trying to find a good hangover cure the next morning when you're already in severe pain and trying not to vomit. Did you know you could do this? As long as you don't do anything silly like binge drinking, mixing your drinks or gulping down too much low-grade alcohol, then this preventative remedy works around 9 times out of 10. How do you do it?

When you drink plenty of alcohol, your body is losing essential vitamins and minerals. Alcohol is a diuretic which means it causes you to expel liquid from your body at a faster rate than you would do normally. The trick is for you to replace these vitamins and minerals (known as electrolytes) as they leave your body.

How do you do this? You take a multivitamin pill right after drinking and before sleeping. But your head should be clear and more alert, with no headache or nausea. You'll definitely feel much better than if you don't take the tablets. Remember to have a big glass of water with your vitamins too, to help to rehydrate your body.

2. Ibuprofen hangover remedy

Normally I'd advice against taking painkillers to cure hangovers. I prefer to recommend only natural hangover remedies and nothing else. But I understand that some hangovers are just too severe and many people have to be active the next day. Some of you have to work and may have an important day. Others may just be in unbearable pain.

What do you do when you feel this way? First of all, never take painkillers right after drinking. Mixing medication with alcohol has health risks and your body may react badly to it. Only take painkillers if you wake up in severe pain and you need to get rid of your headache and nausea very fast.

You can take Ibuprofen to block the pain and reduce nausea, while you recover from your hangover by drinking plenty of liquid and eating food such as eggs (beneficial to your liver) and toast (starch that raises your blood sugar level) with honey (fructose that processes your hangover faster). It's also recommended to get some exercise (walking and fresh air) to improve blood circulation.

3. Eggs and bacon

As discussed earlier; Food is a good hangover cure that works. Generally, for the moderate level of hangover, food can bring you back to life by raising your blood sugar level, diluting the level of alcohol in your blood and helping your body metabolize the alcohol faster. The question is which food?

Don't eat too much when you're hungover. You may feel starving, but eating plates of carbs and French fries can cause you to slump into a digestive meltdown. You'll feel slow, lethargic and not really much better than before. Ideally, you need eggs for their cysteine, which helps to clean up the toxins your body is processing (acetaldehyde).

You need some toast to provide the starch that will raise your blood sugar level and cause you to feel more energetic and less lethargic. You need bacon to provide you with amino acids that help your brain to function better. That's why toast, eggs, and bacon is an excellent hangover remedy.

4. Drinks to help hangover recovery

Certain drinks are great for accelerating our recovery from a bad hangover. Whether you've taken a painkiller to block your headache and nausea or not, drinks are your best way to rehydrate your body, process your hangover faster and flush out the alcohol.

Water on its own may help when you're badly hangover, but it's not ⬜uite enough. Ideally, you should knock back a big tomato juice with salt and pepper. This can be very effective at fixing a bad hangover in a short-term. Cola is fairly effective too, re-hydrating your body and raising your blood sugar level.

5. Home remedies for hangovers

Why venture out into the street when the shops may be closed and when you feel as rough as a badger?

You may even have a good hangover cure at home, in your kitchen cupboard. Home remedies are not just food, drink and natural remedies around your house but they are also what you do with yourself.

Playing golf, taking a walk, taking deep breaths of fresh air, having sex, drinking tea with honey...any combination of these can help you beat a moderate hangover.

Hangover cures to avoid

Just like with anything, there are plenty of myths that circulate about curing hangovers.

1. Tylenol or Paracetamol

I've seen people claiming that taking Tylenol or Paracetamol (also known as Acetaminophen) is a good hangover cure. Some people even have 2 x 500mg tablets right after drinking heavily.

Let me warn you that this is a huge mistake. Acetaminophen is broken down by the liver and adds an additional load on the liver. People who take too much of it in a short time can end up with liver damage. Even the FDA report the liver damage that it can cause.

2. Coffee

Whoever claims that coffee cures hangovers has never really been hangover. Yes, a strong espresso clears your head if you had a few drinks and went to bed late. But for real hangovers, coffee doesn't help at all.

It tightens your headache, appears to dehydrate you even more and finally, leaves you irritable and unable to get back to sleep. People who recommend that coffee fix you up mean well, but they don't know what they're talking about.

3. Hair of the dog

I know hair of the dog as a hangover cure is fun when you're being a bit young and carefree. It appears to work for an hour or two. Then your hangover just hits in again, but slower and for longer.

Getting rid of a hangover is about processing it from your body faster than you would otherwise and replacing what you lost. It's not about giving it more of what makes it hurt. Avoid hair of the dog.

4. Not drinking to avoid hangovers

We've all heard this utter garbage from people claiming they know all about hangovers. "The only way to avoid a hangover is to abstain from drinking."

The whole point in finding a good hangover cure is because you're a drinker. You like a drink. You go to parties, you relax with a drink. So if you're looking for a good hangover cure, the very last thing you want to hear is someone who thinks he knows it all telling you not to drink.

Someone recommending that you don't drink to avoid hangovers is the very last one you want to hear when you wake up hungover. You've already been drinking, so this advice is utterly pointless and useless.

CHAPTER SIX
WHAT TO EAT WHEN YOU HAVE A HANGOVER?

When you have a hangover, you are suffering deeply from a headache, dry mouth, dizziness, and nausea. The biggest problem is that, even though you are nauseous, you need to eat and drink something to make you feel better. Here are some effective food remedies for hangovers.

One common remedy is to drink is more of the "hair of the dog that bit you". This is not really a remedy because it only prolongs the effects of the hangover and you can actually get worse before you get better. Drinking the "hair of the dog" will counteract some of the symptoms in the beginning but, as the liver now has more toxins to process, you are actually making yourself worse.

Another remedy that people often think of is burnt toast. Burnt toast contains burnt carbon in it, but it isn't the same as the activated charcoal found in many over the counter remedies for a hangover. While you certainly can have burnt toast and it will soothe your stomach, there is no benefit to burning it and you can have your toast normally toasted.

This will help soothe your stomach and it will taste good as well.

Black coffee contains caffeine which clamps down on your blood vessels and improves the headache, especially if you take it with acetaminophen. You need to be aware, however, that caffeine is a diuretic, meaning that it causes you a loss of water in your body. Drink plenty of water along with a cup of black coffee and you will have the best of both worlds.

Some people recommend eating fatty foods or fried foods to get rid of a hangover. Fried foods can be irritating to the stomach when you have a hangover so be wary of that problem. Fatty foods, on the other hand, stay in the stomach longer, so when you drink, the absorption of alcohol is slowed down. You will have additional time to absorb and process the byproducts of drinking. It is best to eat the fried or fatty foods during or before drinking so that you can prevent the hangover symptoms from occurring in the first place.

People in the Mediterranean areas of the world take a tablespoonful of olive oil before they drink in order to prevent a hangover.

Once you have the hangover, however, fatty foods won't make a difference.

Fried or boiled eggs give you plenty of energy and also contain a great amount of cysteine that breaks down acetaldehyde in the body. It is acetaldehyde that is one of the toxins left over from drinking. Eggs can help the liver function better and get rid of acetaldehyde along with the liver. So eggs are an excellent choice for a hangover breakfast.

Bananas are touted as good hangover remedies. You eat them after you wake up in the morning. They contain a great many missing electrolytes, including potassium. Sports drinks containing potassium and Kiwi fruit that contain potassium are also good ways to replace the potassium lost by the diuretic effect of alcohol.

Never forget to drink plenty of water before, during and after drinking. It is the best hangover remedy around and will dilute out toxins and give you back the water you lost during your drinking binge.

HANGOVER TIPS

Here are the top 10 hangover tips that could definitely help you on your next night out. The first 5 tips are pretty common; the second 5 tips get into specific nutrients that are known to help hangovers.

Here they are...

1. Drink a lot of water

The effective rule of thumb is to drink a glass of water with every drink or beer. That could be difficult, and cause you to pee lot. At the least, drinking a couple of glasses of water before going to bed can help with the dehydration effect of alcohol.

2. Stay away from mixing alcohols

Stick to one type of alcohol when having drinks. Whether it's just beer, just wine or just whiskey, the second you mix the alcohols you can have some problems. Everyone has that friend who drank a little bit everything one night and was sick as a dog (or maybe that was you).

3. Minimize sweet drinks

An overdose of sugar with a good amount of alcohol is another recipe for disaster. The spike of sugar can have the effect of drinking a Red Bull or two, and then having an energy crash, but it can be twice as worse with alcohol in your system. Next time, minimize the amount those sweet drinks such as Coke and hard liquor, schnapps, imitation flavored margaritas and daiquiris.

4. Monitor your drinking

Going out with and having fun with your friends doesn't mean you have to chug a keg of beer or down a bottle of wine. It's not rocket science to know this tip, but it's a good reminder. And you thank yourself the next morning!

5. Eat a healthy meal before going out

Eating a good meal before going out makes a world of a difference. You won't get as drunk with a full stomach, your body will have the energy to up-keep with the social atmospheres and you'll have some nutrition to ease the effects of alcohol.

The second 5 tips

And now for the second half. Alcohol is known to deplete nutrients from your body, which is assumed to be a major reason for getting hangovers. By simply replacing those nutrients and adding nutrients known to be good for a hangover, you have the best chance to wake up feeling good the next day.

Let's just say that if you utilize these next 5 tips, you have the best chance to not wake up with a hangover. It is best to use these nutrients right before or during drinking, rather than the next day after you already have the hangover.

To continue the list, here are 5 nutrients known to be good for hangovers.

6. Prickly pear

This cactus found mainly in Arizona of the US regions is vastly growing popular because of hangover studies coming out from places like Tulane University Sciences Center in New Orleans. It's no surprise; the Aztecs started cultivating the plant in Mexico in the early sixteenth century for its medicinal purposes.

7. Milk thistle

With strong antioxidant properties and liver-protecting abilities, milk thistle has been used on hangovers for a very long time.

Becky Pugh, from Telegraph, states after testing multiple hangover remedies, "This is by far the best remedy. It eliminated nausea and limited that debilitating tiredness."

8. Vitamin C

Being an important antioxidant, Vitamin C has been shown to reduce the toxic effects of alcohol in the liver, along with speeding up the metabolism of alcohol by the liver. It is also essential to re-hydration of the body.

9. Vitamin B

It is theorized that the depletion of Vitamin B causes a hangover. Either way, vitamin B1 calms your shaky nervous system and helps your weary body break down still-lurking alcohol.

Vitamin B3 (Niacin) helps your digestive system function and promotes a normal appetite. Niacin plays an important role in removing toxic and harmful chemicals from the body and is also effective in improving circulation. And Vitamin B5 helps with fatigue, weakness and possibly headaches.

10. Taurine

This popular natural amino acid coming from the energy drink craze works synergistically with B and C vitamins to help increase the metabolism of the liver, speeding up the detoxification process. It also provides energy, but without the jittery feeling like caffeine.

CONCLUSION

If you have ever wondered what causes hangovers the answer to that question is simply this, hangovers are caused by drinking more alcohol than your body can handle. Even a single alcoholic drink can trigger a hangover for some people. Some may drink heavily and escape a hangover entirely. Generally, however, more than three to five alcoholic drinks for a woman and over five to six for a man will usually result in a hangover. About 75 percent of people who drink alcohol to intoxication will have a hangover the next day.

The effects of hangovers typically begin within several hours after your last drink. Depending on what you drank and how much you drank, you may experience fatigue, thirst, headaches and muscle aches, nausea, vomiting or stomach pain, poor or decreased sleep, sensitivity to light and sound, dizziness or a sense of the room spinning, rapid heartbeat, bloodshot eyes, shakiness, decreased ability to concentrate, mood disturbances, such as depression, anxiety and irritation and more.

Just about anyone who drinks alcohol beverages can experience a hangover. However, some people are more susceptible to hangovers than are others. Research hasn't clearly shown whether light drinkers or heavy drinkers are more likely to experience hangovers.

If you want to avoid or prevent a hangover there a variety of good way to do just that, one would be to eat a good dinner before you go out drinking. Food will absorb some of the alcohol you are going to drink. When you drink choose clear alcohol like light rum, white wine, or vodka or light beer. Continue to eat while you are drinking especially foods higher in fat and carbohydrates, like pretzels or chocolate. This will slow down on the alcohol absorption. Drinking water along with or after every alcoholic beverage will help you to avoid a nasty headache. If you feel a hangover coming on in the morning, eat something and take some Ibuprofen, drink several large glasses of water, and go back to sleep.

However, you can prevent hangovers altogether. Preventing hangovers is as easy as taking a natural supplement before you go out.

Visualize, if you can, simply consuming a natural supplement pill before you drink alcohol that will prevent hangover without any negative side effects what so ever and you have just experienced Goodbye to Hangovers.

www.ingramcontent.com/pod-product-compliance
Lightning Source LLC
Chambersburg PA
CBHW071425220526
45469CB00004B/1431